AF799839

Name:____________________

Medication Allergies:

History at a Glance:
Diagnosis List:

Medication List:

DO NOT RESUSITATE: Check for DNR ☐
(See signature on page 85)

EMERGENCY

Personal Health Record

Introduction

The Personal Health Record & Medical Reference Guide is designed to store your medical history. You or a caregiver can keep a record of medications, allergies, labs, and test results. Keeping track of this information is now simplified. We have included a list of recommended exams, vaccines and tests, along with a Log section, to help you monitor and maintain your own health records and evaluations. This guide is compiled of routine recommendations, your personal physician may have alternate recommendations or schedules based on your personal history.

This Personal Health Record is a summary of your health care. You are now equipped to manage and maintain your medical record. Keeping an updated file will help coordinate your care and reduce the error factor in your medical treatment. This can be especially helpful if you see multiple physicians, rely on family, or other caregivers.

As we have seen, computer hacking, electrical outages, natural disasters, and other unforeseen calamities can and will make electronic medical records inaccessible or unreliable at times. Protect yourself with this simple and portable record.

Table of Contents:

Chapter 1
Emergency Information

This section of the book will provide emergency responders with critical information. By keeping this information up to date vital minutes can be saved in an emergency.

The following chapters will highlight your chronic medical history, including your medication list, allergies, and medical history.

Chapter 1

Emergency
Emergency Information
Medical Information

Personal Contact Information

Name:______________________________________

Address: ___________________________________

City: _____________________ State:______

Zip: _____________________

Telephone Numbers:

Home:(_____) ________ - _____________

Work: (_____) ________ - _____________

Cell: (_____) ________ - _____________

E-Mail: ____________________________________

Secondary Contact Information

Name:______________________________________

Telephone Numbers:

Home:(_____) ________ - _____________

Work: (_____) ________ - _____________

Cell: (_____) ________ - _____________

E-Mail: ____________________________________

Primary Care Physician

Name:______________________________________

Address: ___________________________________

City: _____________________ State:______

Zip: _____________________

Telephone Numbers:

Office: (_____) ________ - _____________

Cell: (_____) ________ - _____________

E-Mail: ____________________________________

Primary Language:____________________________

Marital Status: ☐ Single ☐ Married ☐ Widowed

☐ Divorced ☐ Separated

Religious Affiliation:____________________________

Personal Identification Marks:

☐ Birthmarks ☐ Scars ☐ Tattoos ☐ Piercing

Descriptions and Locations:

____

____

____

____

Living Will: ☐ Yes ☐ No

Organ / Tissue Donor: ☐ Yes ☐ No

Blood Type: ____________

Allergies:☐ Yes (See Chapter 3) ☐ No

Durable Power of Attorney

Name:____

Address:______________________________________

City: ____________________ State:______

Zip: ____________________

Telephone Numbers:

Home:(_____) __________ - ____________________

Work:(_____) __________ - ____________________

Cell: (_____) __________ - ____________________

E-Mail____

Health Insurance

Medicare Number:________________________

Telephone: (_____) _________ - ________________

Primary Insurance Company:

____

Identification Number: _________________________
Group Number:_______________________________

Telephone: (_____) _________ - ________________

Effective Date _____/_____/_______
Cancellation Date _____/_____/_______

Secondary Insurance Company:

____

Identification Number: _________________________
Group Number:_______________________________

Telephone: (_____) _________ - ________________

Effective Date _____/_____/_______
Cancellation Date _____/_____/_______

Dental Insurance Company:

____

Identification Number: _________________________
Group Number:_______________________________

Telephone: (_____) _________ - ________________

Effective Date _____/_____/_______
Cancellation Date _____/_____/_______

List of Doctors and Facilities

Primary Care:

____

Address:_______________________________________

City: ___________________ State_____________
Zip:___________________

Telephone: (_____) _________ - _________________

Pharmacy:

____

Address:_______________________________________

City: ___________________ State:_____________
Zip: ___________________

Telephone: (_____) _________ - _________________

Hospital Name:_______________________________

Address:_______________________________________

City: ___________________ State: ______________
Zip: ___________________

Telephone: (_____) _________ - _________________

Specialists:

Dr.______________________________

Specialty:______________________________

Phone: (_____) ______ - ________

Dr.______________________________

Specialty:______________________________

Phone: (_____) ______ - ________

Dr.______________________________

Specialty:______________________________

Phone: (_____) ______ - ________

Dr.______________________________

Specialty:______________________________

Phone: (_____) ______ - ________

Dr.______________________________

Specialty:______________________________

Phone: (_____) ______ - ________

Specialists:

Dr.______________________________

Specialty:_____________________________

Phone: (_____) ______ - ________

Dr.______________________________

Specialty:_____________________________

Phone: (_____) ______ - ________

Dr.______________________________

Specialty:_____________________________

Phone: (_____) ______ - ________

Dr.______________________________

Specialty:_____________________________

Phone: (_____) ______ - ________

Dr.______________________________

Specialty:_____________________________

Phone: (_____) ______ - ________

Secondary Hospital:______________________________

Address:____

City: ___________________ State: ____________
Zip: ___________________

Telephone: (____) _________ - _________________

Secondary Pharmacy _____________________________

Address:____

City: ___________________ State: ______________
Zip: ___________________

Telephone: (____) _________ - __________________

Dentist Name: ________________________________

Address:____

City: ___________________ State: ______________
Zip: ___________________

Telephone: (____) _________ - ________________

Orthodontist Name: ______________________________

Address:____

City: ___________________ State: ______________
Zip: ___________________

Telephone: (____) _________ - ________________

Chapter 2
Medication List

This list will help coordinate your care with all of your doctors and care givers. It will save time, improve care, and reduce errors. Keep it current.

If a medication is stopped due to side effects, add a brief note about this in the "Notes" section following your list.

Example:

Medication	Strength	Number Per Day
Medication name	*# mg.*	*2*

☐ Check box if medication is stopped or changed and rewrite new instructions on a new line.

Medication / Supplements	Strength	Number Per Day

☐ ______________________________

☐ ______________________________

☐ ______________________________

☐ ______________________________

☐ ______________________________

☐ ______________________________

☐ ______________________________

Medication / Supplements	Strength	Number Per Day
☐		
☐		
☐		
☐		
☐		
☐		
☐		
☐		
☐		
☐		
☐		
☐		
☐		
☐		
☐		

Medication / Supplements	Strength	Number Per Day
☐		
☐		
☐		
☐		
☐		
☐		
☐		
☐		
☐		
☐		
☐		
☐		
☐		
☐		
☐		

Medication / Supplements	Strength	Number Per Day
☐		
☐		
☐		
☐		
☐		
☐		
☐		
☐		
☐		
☐		
☐		
☐		
☐		
☐		

Chapter 3
Allergies

This section addresses allergies that are life threatening and also those that are of a nuisance nature. A checklist of common allergies, including various foods, is provided to improve awareness and one's quality of life.

Mark box with check ☑ if mild allergy.
Mark box with X ☒ if severe allergy.

Medications:

- ☐ Acetaminophen
- ☐ Amoxicillin
- ☐ Ampicillin
- ☐ Aspirin
- ☐ Ciprofloxin.
- ☐ Codeine
- ☐ Demerol
- ☐ Erythromycin
- ☐ Ibuprofen
- ☐ Iodine
- ☐ Penicillin
- ☐ Sulfa
- ☐ Tetracycline

Other:____

____

Seasonal Inhalants:

☐ Grasses ☐ Trees ☐ Weeds

Other:______________________________

Non-seasonal Inhalants:

- ☐ Animals
- ☐ Latex
- ☐ Chemicals
- ☐ House/Dust Mites
- ☐ Insects
- ☐ Molds

Other:______________________________

History of Food Allergy:

☐ Anaphylaxis

Notes:

Allergies

Chapter 4
Medical History

A patient's past medical history often gives insights into current symptoms and future risks.

This may help your doctors avoid errors and delays in treatment.

If you change physicians or see a specialist for any reason this section provides an important picture of your past health issues.

Keeping this section current may also reduce unnecessary or repeat testing. It will help your physicians coordinate your care in a more effective and efficient manner.

Chapter 4
Medical History

Diagnosis: **Date of onset**
Notes:

Diagnosis: ______________________________ /____/____
Notes:____

____

Diagnosis: ______________________________ /____/____
Notes:____

____

Diagnosis: ______________________________ /____/____
Notes:____

____

Diagnosis: ______________________________ /____/____
Notes:____

____

Diagnosis: ______________________________ /____/____
Notes:____

____

Diagnosis: ______________________________ /____/____
Notes:____

____

Diagnosis: ______________________________ /____/____
Notes:____

____

Diagnosis: ______________________/____/____
Notes:____________________________________

____

Diagnosis: ______________________/____/____
Notes:____________________________________

____

Diagnosis: ______________________/____/____
Notes:____________________________________

____

Diagnosis: ______________________/____/____
Notes:____________________________________

____

Diagnosis: ______________________/____/____
Notes:____________________________________

____

Diagnosis: ______________________/____/____
Notes:____________________________________

____

Diagnosis: ______________________/____/____
Notes:____________________________________

____

Diagnosis: ______________________/____/____
Notes:____________________________________

____

Diagnosis: ______________________/____/____
Notes:____________________________________

____

Diagnosis: ______________________________/____/____
Notes:____

____

Diagnosis: ______________________________/____/____
Notes:____

____

Diagnosis: ______________________________/____/____
Notes:____

____

Diagnosis: ______________________________/____/____
Notes:____

____

Diagnosis: ______________________________/____/____
Notes:____

____

Diagnosis: ______________________________/____/____
Notes:____

____

Diagnosis: ______________________________/____/____
Notes:____

____

Diagnosis: ______________________________/____/____
Notes:____

____

Diagnosis: ______________________________/____/____
Notes:____

____

Chapter 5
Hospitalization, Surgery, Injury History

The following section will serve as a reference for previous hospitalizations, surgeries, or injuries. This gives insight to the nature and severity of previous problems.

- Cardiovascular (Heart / Circulation)
- Endocrine (Diabetes / Thyroid / Other glands)
- GI Tract (Esophagus / Stomach / Intestine / Colon / Rectum / Gallbladder)
- Hematology (Blood disorders / Anemia)
- Hepatology (Liver)
- Immunology (Immune disorders)
- Infectious Disease
- Nephrology (Kidneys)
- Neurology / Neurosurgery (Brain / Nerves)
- OB/GYN (Female Health)
- Oncology (Cancer)
- Ophthalmology (Eyes)
- Orthopedics (Bones / Musculoskeletal / Injuries)
- Otolaryngology (Ears / Nose / Throat)
- Plastic Surgery (Reconstructive / Cosmetic)
- Podiatry (Foot)
- Psychiatry (Mental Health)
- Pulmonology (Lungs)
- Rheumatology (Joints)
- Transplant Surgery (Organs)
- Urology (Genitourinary Tract – Kidneys / Bladder / Prostate / External organs)

Chapter 5

Hospitalization, Surgery, Injury History

Date / Reason / Outcome:______________________________

____

____

____

____

Date / Reason / Outcome:______________________________

____

____

____

____

Date / Reason / Outcome:______________________________

____

____

____

____

Date / Reason / Outcome:______________________________

____

____

____

____

Date / Reason / Outcome:______________________________

____

____

____

____

Date / Reason / Outcome:________________________________

____

____

____

____

Date / Reason / Outcome:________________________________

____

____

____

____

Date / Reason / Outcome:________________________________

____

____

____

____

Date / Reason / Outcome:________________________________

____

____

____

____

Date / Reason / Outcome:________________________________

____

____

____

____

Date / Reason / Outcome:________________________________

____

____

____

____

Date / Reason / Outcome:________________________

Date / Reason / Outcome:________________________

Date / Reason / Outcome:________________________

Date / Reason / Outcome:________________________

Date / Reason / Outcome:________________________

Date / Reason / Outcome:________________________

Chapter 6
Issues: Female and Male

This section addresses male and female organ health. Additionally, it includes information related to reproductive health history.

There is a list of additional issues related to reproductive health in the Chapter 12 **Discussions to Have with Your Doctor** section.

Male:
Diagnosis: **Date of onset**
Notes:

☐ ☐BPH (Large Prostate) ____/____/____
Notes:____
____

☐ ☐Loss of Libido ____/____/____
Notes:____
____

☐ ☐Prostate Cancer ____/____/____
Notes:____
____

☐ ☐Erectile Dysfunction ____/____/____
Notes:____
____

☐ ☐Other *(Please List)* ____/____/____
Notes:____
____

☐ ☐Other *(Please List)* ____/____/____
Notes:____
____

Chapter 6
Issues: Female

Diagnosis: **Date of onset**

☐ Age 1st Menstrual Period ____/____/____
☐ Irregular Periods ____/____/____
☐ Heavy Menstrual Periods ____/____/____
☐ Painful Periods ____/____/____

☐ Ovarian Cysts ____/____/____
☐ Endometriosis ____/____/____
☐ Fibroids ____/____/____
☐ PMS ____/____/____
☐ Fibrocystic Breast ____/____/____
☐ Infertility ____/____/____
☐ Loss of Libido ____/____/____
☐ Recurrent UTI ____/____/____
☐ Chronic Yeast Infection ____/____/____

☐ Pregnancies #______

☐ Miscarriages #______

☐ Other ______

Notes:

____

____

____

____

Female Log of Studies and Tests

Pap Smear Log

Pap smear Date	Result	Breast Exam
___/___/___	______________	No☐ Yes☐
___/___/___	______________	No☐ Yes☐
___/___/___	______________	No☐ Yes☐
___/___/___	______________	No☐ Yes☐
___/___/___	______________	No☐ Yes☐
___/___/___	______________	No☐ Yes☐
___/___/___	______________	No☐ Yes☐

Mammogram Date: ___/___/______
Result: ___________________________________
Follow up Due Date: ___/___/______

Mammogram Date: ___/___/______
Result: ___________________________________
Follow up Due Date: ___/___/______

Mammogram Date: ___/___/______
Result: ___________________________________
Follow up Due Date: ___/___/______

Mammogram Date: ___/___/______
Result: ___________________________________
Follow up Due Date: ___/___/______

Notes:

____

____

____

____

Female:

Bone density Date: ___/___/______
Result: __________________________________
Follow up Due Date: ___/___/______

Bone density Date: ___/___/______
Result: __________________________________
Follow up Due Date: ___/___/______

Bone density Date: ___/___/______
Result: __________________________________
Follow up Due Date: ___/___/______

First Day of Last Menstrual Period (LMP)

Date	Heavy	Med	Light
___/___/___	☐	☐	☐
___/___/___	☐	☐	☐
___/___/___	☐	☐	☐
___/___/___	☐	☐	☐
___/___/___	☐	☐	☐
___/___/___	☐	☐	☐
___/___/___	☐	☐	☐
___/___/___	☐	☐	☐
___/___/___	☐	☐	☐
___/___/___	☐	☐	☐
___/___/___	☐	☐	☐
___/___/___	☐	☐	☐
___/___/___	☐	☐	☐
___/___/___	☐	☐	☐

Chapter 7

Health Maintenance Schedule

This is a list of current recommended tests and screens. This should be used as a guideline. Your personal physician may recommend a different schedule based on your personal or family history.

For example, based on family history or symptoms, some people may require a colonoscopy before the age of forty-five, and may require an annual follow up colonoscopy.

Comprehensive Physical exam	18-65+ yrs. - Annually
Periodic physicals	18-65+ yrs. - Annually And Labs or per physician
Blood pressure	18-65+ yrs. Every visit
Weight	18-65+ yrs. Every visit
Cholesterol screening	18-65 yrs. 1-5 years 65+ yrs. - Annually or per physician
Colon Cancer screening	
Fecal / blood test	50-65+ yrs. Annually
Sigmoidoscopy	50-65+ yrs. 3-5 yrs.
Colonoscopy	45-65+ yrs. 5-10 yrs.
Eye/Vision examination	1-3 yrs.
Glaucoma testing	65+ yrs. Annually
Screening for depression	18-65+ yrs. 1-3 yrs.

Chapter 7
Health Maintenance Schedule

Males Only:	**Age:**	**When:**
Testicular exam	18+ yrs.	Self exam monthly
Physical exam	18+ yrs.	Annually
STD/STI Panel	Discuss with physician	

Females Only:	**Age:**	**When:**
Clinical breast exam	18+ yrs.	Annually Self exam monthly
Mammography	40+ yrs.	Annually / Biannual
Osteoporosis Screening	65 + yrs.	Every 2yrs
(For some age 50, discuss with MD)		
Pap smear		Annually or per MD
Pelvic Exam		Annually
STD/STI Panel	Discuss with physician	

Notes:____

Chapter 8

Recommended Immunizations

This is the current list of recommend immunizations. It is important to keep it updated, as some immunizations require periodic boosters. It is noteworthy, that some schools and some professions may mandate proof of immunization.

If the dates of your vaccinations are no longer available, immunity titres can be obtained. These are lab tests that document immunity status or the need for a booster. They can be used as a substitute on forms when the actual proof of immunization dates are not available or have been lost.

The SARS-CoV-2 (COVID-19) virus pandemic has devastated global health and has severed societal, cultural, and political norms. The impact of this pandemic has shocked entire nations, disrupted organizations, and divided families. The specter of death, illness, and long COVID has left in its wake an extraordinary degree of suffering. A significant number of those, untouched by the virus itself, were left fighting the effects of isolation and enduring depression.

Some survival correlations have been noted. Though not based on a double-blind study, data suggests that people who complete 12,000 steps per day are less likely to suffer severe COVID infections compared to those who do 4,000 steps or fewer per day. Additionally, it suggests that individuals with a vitamin D deficiency are more prone to severe COVID infections than those in the normal range. While the long-term effects of COVID vaccines are still being studied, there is a significant correlation between improved overall health and the use of COVID vaccines at this point.

COVID-19 / SARS
Vaccination Record

Date(s) Immunization Received:

____________________ ____________________
____________________ ____________________
____________________ ____________________
____________________ ____________________
____________________ ____________________

Date(s) of Infection: Long Covid Symptoms? (Y/N)

_______________ ______________________________
_______________ ______________________________
_______________ ______________________________
_______________ ______________________________
_______________ ______________________________

Notes:

____
____
____
____
____

****************COVID19 UPDATE****************

May 2023, the U.S. Food and Drug Administration approved the oral antiviral Paxlovid (nirmatrelvir tablets and ritonavir tablets, co-packaged for oral use) for the treatment of mild-to-moderate COVID-19 in adults who are at high risk for progression to severe COVID-19, including hospitalization or death. Paxlovid is the fourth drug, and first oral antiviral pill, approved by the FDA to treat COVID-19 in adults. This medication may provide additional protection to individuals at high risk and the unvaccinated who have already contracted the virus.

****

Chapter 8
Recommended Immunizations

Vaccination		Date Received
Hepatitis A/B	(HepA/B#1)	____________
	(HepA/B#2)	____________
	(HepA/B#3)	____________
Diphtheria/ Tetanus/ Pertussis	(DTaP#1)	____________
	(DTaP#2)	____________
	(DTaP#3)	____________
	(DTap#4)	____________
	(DTaP#5)	____________
Haemophilus/ Influenza/type b	(Hib#1)	____________
	(Hib#2)	____________
	(Hib#3)	____________
	(Hib#4)	____________
Inactivated/ Poliovirus	(IPV#1)	____________
	(IPV#2)	____________
	(IPV#3)	____________
	(IPV#4)	____________
Pneumococcal/ Conjugate	(PCV#1)	____________
	(PCV#2)	____________
	(PCV#3)	____________
HPV	(1)	____________
	(2)	____________
	(3)	____________
Meningitis		____________

Vaccination	Date Received
Measles/Mumps/ (MMR#1)	______________
Rubella (MMR#2)	______________
Varicella	______________
Pneumococcal	______________
	______________

This vaccination is repeated every 7-10 years:

DTaP / Tetanus (Td)	______________
	______________

This vaccination is issued on an individual basis

Influenza	______________
	______________
	______________
Shingles / Varicella	______________

Recommended Travel Immunizations

Vaccination	Date Received
Dengue Fever	______________
Gamma Globulin	______________
Hepatitis A/B	______________
Japanese Encephalitis Vaccine	______________
Rabies Vaccine	______________
Typhoid Fever	______________
Yellow Fever	______________
RSV (Respiratory Syncytial Virus)	______________
Malaria Prophylaxis	______________
Other	______________

____

____

____

Chapter 9
Log of Studies and Tests

Many studies and tests are performed for routine health screening. Many are done to diagnose a particular problem. Use these logs to remain current with screening tests and to record any results of studies, which may help with diagnosis and treatment planning.

This is your lifeline to monitoring your studies and test results. By maintaining your logs you can track trends as they occur. This will allow you and your doctors to make adjustments as needed. It also allows you to track your improvements.

Use this section to help you achieve your long-term health goals. For example, achieving a healthy weight, blood pressure or sugar level may dramatically reduce future health problems and the hardships they cause.

If you are being treated for high blood pressure, we recommend that you log an average weekly blood pressure in the following section. This will allow you to monitor trends and the effectiveness of your treatment. We have included additional lines and a notes section to log any significant peaks or drops in your blood pressure. Use the notes section to describe any symptoms that may have been associated with these changes.

Chapter 9
Log of Studies and Tests

Weight Log and Blood Pressure Log

Date:	Weight	Blood Pressure
___/___/___	________	________
___/___/___	________	________
___/___/___	________	________
___/___/___	________	________
___/___/___	________	________
___/___/___	________	________
___/___/___	________	________
___/___/___	________	________
___/___/___	________	________
___/___/___	________	________
___/___/___	________	________
___/___/___	________	________
___/___/___	________	________
___/___/___	________	________
___/___/___	________	________
___/___/___	________	________
___/___/___	________	________
___/___/___	________	________
___/___/___	________	________
___/___/___	________	________
___/___/___	________	________
___/___/___	________	________
___/___/___	________	________
___/___/___	________	________
___/___/___	________	________

Date:	Weight	Blood Pressure
____/____/____	__________	__________
____/____/____	__________	__________
____/____/____	__________	__________
____/____/____	__________	__________
____/____/____	__________	__________
____/____/____	__________	__________
____/____/____	__________	__________
____/____/____	__________	__________
____/____/____	__________	__________
____/____/____	__________	__________
____/____/____	__________	__________
____/____/____	__________	__________
____/____/____	__________	__________
____/____/____	__________	__________
____/____/____	__________	__________
____/____/____	__________	__________
____/____/____	__________	__________
____/____/____	__________	__________
____/____/____	__________	__________
____/____/____	__________	__________
____/____/____	__________	__________
____/____/____	__________	__________
____/____/____	__________	__________
____/____/____	__________	__________
____/____/____	__________	__________
____/____/____	__________	__________
____/____/____	__________	__________
____/____/____	__________	__________
____/____/____	__________	__________
____/____/____	__________	__________

Date:	Weight	Blood Pressure
___/___/___	________	________
___/___/___	________	________
___/___/___	________	________
___/___/___	________	________
___/___/___	________	________
___/___/___	________	________
___/___/___	________	________
___/___/___	________	________
___/___/___	________	________
___/___/___	________	________
___/___/___	________	________
___/___/___	________	________
___/___/___	________	________
___/___/___	________	________
___/___/___	________	________
___/___/___	________	________
___/___/___	________	________
___/___/___	________	________
___/___/___	________	________
___/___/___	________	________
___/___/___	________	________
___/___/___	________	________
___/___/___	________	________
___/___/___	________	________
___/___/___	________	________
___/___/___	________	________
___/___/___	________	________
___/___/___	________	________
___/___/___	________	________
___/___/___	________	________

Notes:

Log of Studies and Tests

Type of Study / Date:______________________________
Results:____

Follow up due date:________________________________

Type of Study / Date:______________________________
Results:____

Follow up due date:________________________________

Type of Study / Date:______________________________
Results:____

Follow up due date:________________________________

Type of Study / Date:______________________________
Results:____

Follow up due date:________________________________

Type of Study / Date:______________________________
Results:____

Follow up due date:________________________________

Type of Study / Date:____________________________
Results:______________________________________

____

____

Follow up due date:______________________________

Type of Study / Date:____________________________
Results:______________________________________

____

____

Follow up due date:______________________________

Type of Study / Date:____________________________
Results:______________________________________

____

____

Follow up due date:______________________________

Type of Study / Date:____________________________
Results:______________________________________

____

____

Follow up due date:______________________________

Type of Study / Date:____________________________
Results:______________________________________

____

____

Follow up due date:______________________________

Type of Study / Date:____________________________
Results:______________________________________

____

____

Follow up due date:______________________________

Blood Tests

Type of Test ________ Date: ___/___/_____
Result: ______________________________
Follow up Due Date: ___/___/______

________________________ Date: ___/___/_____
Result: ______________________________
Follow up Due Date: ___/___/______

________________________ Date: ___/____/_____
Result: ______________________________
Follow up Due Date: ___/___/______

________________________ Date: ___/___/_____
Result: ______________________________
Follow up Due Date: ___/___/______

________________________ Date: ___/___/_____
Result: ______________________________
Follow up Due Date: ___/___/______

________________________ Date: ___/___/_____
Result: ______________________________
Follow up Due Date: ___/___/______

________________________ Date: ___/____/_____
Result: ______________________________
Follow up Due Date: ___/___/______

________________________ Date: ___/___/_____
Result: ______________________________
Follow up Due Date: ___/___/______

Blood Tests

__________________________ Date: ___/___/_____
Result: _______________________________________
Follow up Due Date: ___/___/______

__________________________ Date: ___/___/_____
Result: _______________________________________
Follow up Due Date: ___/___/______

__________________________ Date: ___/____/____
Result: _______________________________________
Follow up Due Date: ___/___/______

__________________________ Date: ___/___/_____
Result: _______________________________________
Follow up Due Date: ___/___/______

__________________________ Date: ___/___/_____
Result: _______________________________________
Follow up Due Date: ___/___/______

__________________________ Date: ___/___/_____
Result: _______________________________________
Follow up Due Date: ___/___/______

__________________________ Date: ___/____/____
Result: _______________________________________
Follow up Due Date: ___/___/______

__________________________ Date: ___/___/_____
Result: _______________________________________
Follow up Due Date: ___/___/______

Blood Tests

________________________ Date: ___/___/_____
Result: ____________________________________
Follow up Due Date: ___/___/______

________________________ Date: ___/___/_____
Result: ____________________________________
Follow up Due Date: ___/___/______

________________________ Date: ___/____/____
Result: ____________________________________
Follow up Due Date: ___/___/______

________________________ Date: ___/___/_____
Result: ____________________________________
Follow up Due Date: ___/___/______

________________________ Date: ___/___/_____
Result: ____________________________________
Follow up Due Date: ___/___/______

________________________ Date: ___/___/_____
Result: ____________________________________
Follow up Due Date: ___/___/______

________________________ Date: ___/____/____
Result: ____________________________________
Follow up Due Date: ___/___/______

________________________ Date: ___/___/_____
Result: ____________________________________
Follow up Due Date: ___/___/______

Blood Tests

_______________________ Date: ___/___/_____
Result: __________________________________
Follow up Due Date: ___/___/______

_______________________ Date: ___/___/_____
Result: __________________________________
Follow up Due Date: ___/___/______

_______________________ Date: ___/____/____
Result: __________________________________
Follow up Due Date: ___/___/______

_______________________ Date: ___/___/_____
Result: __________________________________
Follow up Due Date: ___/___/______

Cancer Screening Tests

Type:____________________ Date: ___/___/_____
Result: ____________________________________
____
____
____
____
____

Type:____________________ Date: ___/___/_____
Result: ____________________________________
____
____
____
____
____

Cholesterol and Lipids

Date:	Total Cholest.	TG	HDL	LDL
___/___/___	________	____	____	____
	LDL-PN-______	IR-______		
___/___/___	________	____	____	____
	LDL-PN-______	IR-______		
___/___/___	________	____	____	____
	LDL-PN-______	IR-______		
___/___/___	________	____	____	____
	LDL-PN-______	IR-______		
___/___/___	________	____	____	____
	LDL-PN-______	IR-______		

Notes:____

TG = Triglycerides

LDL-PN = LDL Particle Number

IR = Insulin Resistance Score

Diabetes:

It is important to track blood glucose levels on a regular basis. Your physician will advise you on how often you should check your levels at home. Most glucometers now include an *average glucose* reading. Use the following chart to monitor your monthly average and periodic HgA1c levels.

Date:	Glucose (Monthly Average)	HgA1c
___/___/___		
___/___/___		
___/___/___		
___/___/___		
___/___/___		
___/___/___		
___/___/___		
___/___/___		
___/___/___		
___/___/___		
___/___/___		
___/___/___		

Notes:

Chapter 10
Visits:
Questions & Recommendations

Use this section to prepare for your appointment with the doctor. It will help the doctor understand your problems or concerns. It will help you to remember the doctors' recommendations. This section is especially important if care givers / family members are helping with your care. It provides a record for those trying to coordinate your health care needs. Maintaining this section can reduce confusion, errors, and mistakes. It also reduces all of the "Oops, I forgot to ask the doctor about…" scenarios.

Chapter 10

Doctor Visits: Questions & Recommendations

Date of Office Visit ____/____/____

Questions:____

Recommendations:____________________________________

Date of Office Visit ____/____/____

Questions:____

Recommendations:____________________________________

Date of Office Visit ____/____/____

Questions:____

Recommendations:____

Date of Office Visit ____/____/____

Questions:____

Recommendations:____

Date of Office Visit ____/____/____

Questions:

Recommendations:

Date of Office Visit ____/____/____

Questions:

Recommendations:

Date of Office Visit ____/____/____

Questions:____

Recommendations:__________________________________

Date of Office Visit ____/____/____

Questions:____

Recommendations:__________________________________

Date of Office Visit ____/____/____

Questions:____

Recommendations:__________________________________

Date of Office Visit ____/____/____

Questions:____

Recommendations:__________________________________

Date of Office Visit ____/____/____

Questions:

Recommendations:

Date of Office Visit ____/____/____

Questions:

Recommendations:

Date of Office Visit ____/____/____

Questions:____

Recommendations:__________________________________

Date of Office Visit ____/____/____

Questions:____

Recommendations:__________________________________

Date of Office Visit ____/____/____

Questions:____

Recommendations:________________________________

Date of Office Visit ____/____/____

Questions:____

Recommendations:________________________________

Notes:

Chapter 11

Family Medical History/Heredity

Some diseases are inherited. This section will help focus medical attention on those specific risks in your family. It may tell your doctor what test to order. Early detection may save your life. Specific lifestyle changes, tests or treatments may help avoid some of the illnesses of your ancestors. Some tests are available for cancer screening.

Genetic testing is under development to provide more specific information. While some of these tests are generally reliable, others need further evaluation. Before drawing conclusions on any of these test results it may be necessary to consult a Genetic Counselor.

Appendix 1 is included as a reference.

Genetic Test Results (DNA): ____________________

____

____

____

____

____

____

____

____

____

____

____

____

____

____

Chapter 11
Family Medical History/Heredity

Check box if family history and list on line family member affected. May abbreviate family members: F (father), M (mother), B (brother), S (sister), PGF / PGM(paternal grandfather/grandmother) and MGF/ MGM (maternal grandfather/grandmother).

☐ Arthritis (Type) ______________________________

☐ Cancer (Type) ______________________________

☐ Diabetes ______________________________

☐ Headaches ______________________________

☐ Heart Disease (Type)______________________________

☐ Hematological Disease (Type) ______________________________

☐ High Blood Pressure ______________________________

☐ Kidney Disease (Type) ______________________________

☐ Mental Health (Type) ______________________________

☐ Neurological (Type) ______________________________

☐ Osteoporosis ______________________________

☐ Seizures ______________________________

☐ Stroke______________________________

☐ Thyroid Disease (Type) ______________________________

☐ Other: ______________________________

____

____

____

Additional Notes Page 67

Chapter 12

Discussions to Have with Your Doctor

Lifestyle/Diet/Exercise & Prevention

When it's your life at stake, *an ounce of prevention* is worth more than *a pound of cure.* The following list of discussions will apply differently to each individual. This section is intended as a checklist. Do not be embarrassed to bring up any of these topics with your doctor. Your doctor is there to help you and understands your need for privacy.

Female:

- Breast self-exam
- Osteoporosis Prevention

Pregnancy:

- Prenatal Care
- Folate / Prenatal Supplements

Males:

- Testicular self-exam
- Discuss PSA (Prostate Specific Antigen)
- Erectile Dysfunction

Sexual Health:

- Reproductive Health/Libido
- Contraception Options
- Sexuality/STIs (STDs)
- Sexual Dysfunction
- Sexual Concerns

Diet and Exercise

Make a commitment to yourself to monitor and maintain a healthy diet and regular exercise program. This contract with yourself may be the single most important health decision that you make.

Diet

Caffeine
Calorie/ Fat/ Salt/ Sugar/ Gluten intake
Diet Supplements / Vitamins
Eating Disorders
Fast foods/Comfort foods
Vegetarian
Weight gain/loss
Other

Exercise:

Frequency
Types of Activity
Body Image concerns

Addictions:

Alcohol/ Tobacco/ Substance Abuse
Gambling/ Sex
Other

Health Issues to Think About

Aspirin use for Prevention of Cardiovascular events
Dental Health
Hearing/ Vision Assessments
Injury and Fall Prevention
Lifetime medic alerts
Living Will (See Medical Forms, Appendix 3)

Alternative Treatment Options
Medications / Diet / Lifestyles
Medication Side Effects

Prevention and Safety:
Medical ID Bracelet:
Seatbelt use
Helmet use for bikes or sports
Smoke detector in home
Carbon monoxide detector in home
Fire extinguisher in home
Water heater temperature check

Sleep quality
Fatigue
Snoring
Memory loss

Occupational Exposure
- Toxic fumes or chemicals
- Radiation
- Excessive heat or cold
- Excessive noise

Equipment maintenance and safety
for auto, hobbies, and sports

Travel: visit www.CDC.gov for immunization and health safety recommendations prior to overseas travel. Also visit www.state.gov for safety recommendations when traveling to foreign countries.

Notes:

Appendix 1: Hereditary Conditions

Albinism
Alzheimer's disease
Becker's muscular dystrophy
Canavan disease
Charcot-Marie-Tooth disease
Chronic myelogenous leukemia
Clinical thalassemia
Color blindness
Congenital cataracts
Cri du chat syndrome (missing chromosome)
Crigler-Najjar syndrome
Cystic fibrosis
Duchenne muscular dystrophy
Ellis-van Creveld syndrome
Facioscapulohumeral muscular dystrophy
Familial dysbetalipo-proteinemia
Familial hypercholesterolemia
Familial hypertriglyceridemia
Familial tremor
Fragile X syndrome
G-6-PD deficiency
Galactosemia
Gaucher's disease-type 1
Hemochromatosis
Hemophilia A
Hereditary amyloidosis
Hereditary elliptocytosis
Huntington's disease
Incontentia pigmenti (Bloch-Sulzberger syndrome)
Klinefelter syndrome (extra X chromosome)
Krabbe's disease
Marfan syndrome

Appendix 1: Medical History

Cardiovascular:

Atherosclerosis
Cardiomyopathy
Chest Pain / Angina
Congestive Heart Failure
Coronary Heart Disease
Dizziness
Endocarditis
Heart Attack
High Blood Pressure
Irregular Heartbeat / Arrhythmia
Low Blood Pressure
Peripheral Vascular Disease
Poor Circulation
Rapid Heartbeat
Swelling of Ankles/Feet / Edema
Valvular Disease
Varicose Veins

Pulmonary:

Asthma
Breathing Pain
Chest Tightness
Chronic Bronchitis
COPD (Chronic Obstructive Pulmonary Disease)
Cough
Emphysema
Interstitial Pulmonary
Pulmonary Embolism
Pulmonary Hypertension
Shortness in Breath
Sleep Apnea

Appendix 2: Medical History

Neurological:

Carpal Tunnel Syndrome
Cerebellar Dysfunction
Dizziness
Double Vision
Drop Attacks
Headaches
Neuropathy
Problems Swallowing
Seizure Disorder
Stroke
TIA (Transient Ischemic Attack)

Brain Syndromes:

Brain Tumor
Domestic Violence
Falling down
Head Trauma
Hematoma / Hemorrhage
Hydrocephalus
Infections
Lack of Oxygen (Anoxia)
Motor Vehicle Accident
Ruptured Aneurysm
Seizures
Stroke

Appendix 2: Medical History

Endocrine:

Adrenal Insufficiency
Changes in Hair, Nails or Skin
Cushing's Disease
Diabetes Mellitus
Frequent Day/Night Urination
Hot Flashes
Irregular Menstrual Periods
Menopause
Osteoporosis
Pituitary Tumor
Polycystic Ovary
Excessive Thirst
Thyroid Disease
Weight Gain
Weight Loss

Appendix 2: Medical History

Gastrointestinal:

Abdominal Pain
Bad Breath, Halitosis
Colitis
Colon Polyps
Constipation
Diarrhea
Diverticulosis
Esophagitis
Esophageal Strictures
Gas, Flatulence
Gastritis
Gastroesophageal Disease
Gastrointestinal Bleed
Inflammatory Bowel Disease
Irritable Bowel Syndrome
Nausea/ Vomiting
Pancreatitis
Peptic Ulcer Disease

Infectious Disease:

Cellulitis
Hepatitis A, B, or C
Immune Disorder
Strep Infection
Tuberculosis/ PPD+

Appendix 2: Medical History

Cancer or Blood Disorders:

Anemia
Bleeding Disorders
Blood Clots
Bone
Brain
Breast
Cervical
Colon
Leukemia
Lung
Lymphoma
Melanoma
Ovarian
Prostate
Skin
Thyroid

Rheumatology:

Ankylosing Spondylitis
Fibromyalgia
Gout
Lupus
Osteoarthritis
Psoriatic Arthritis
Rheumatoid Arthritis
Sarcoidosis
Scleroderma
Sjogren's Syndrome

Appendix 2: Medical History

Mental Health:

ADD/ADHD
Anorexia or Bulimia
Anxiety/Stress
Delusional Thought Disorder
Depression
Manic-Depressive
Obsessive Compulsive Disorder
Panic Attacks
Psychosis
Schizophrenia

Musculoskeletal

Chronic Pain
Carpal Tunnel Syndrome
Chronic Fatigue Syndrome
Muscular Dystrophies
Orthopedic Disorders
Weakness
Other *(Please List)*

Appendix 2: Medical Forms

This appendix includes healthcare related legal forms.

Living Will / Advance Directive
The Living Will and Advance Directive allow you to specify your instructions in the event that you are otherwise incapacitated and unable to give informed consent.
For example, you may wish to decline the use of cardiopulmonary resuscitation or feeding tubes if it is determined by your physician that such measures will serve only to prolong the suffering from an incurable or terminal illness.

Organ Donation
This form confirms your instructions to donate any or all of your organs upon death.

Durable Power of Attorney
Use this to indicate the person, or alternate, who will direct healthcare decisions on your behalf in the event that you are unable to do so. Ideally, discuss this decision and the specifics of your Living Will/ Advance Directive with this person in advance.

DO NOT RESUSCITATE ORDER
This form, and the related Limited Resuscitation Order, allows you to specify the use, or nonuse, of resuscitation techniques in the event that life-sustaining measures become necessary.

These forms cover the basics. For more comprehensive instructions consult an attorney.

Living Will

I want the person I have appointed, my doctors, my family, and others to be guided by the decision I have made below:

These are my wishes for my future medical care if there ever comes a time when I can't make these decisions for myself:

These are my wishes if I have a terminal condition or persistent vegetative state:

Life Sustaining Treatments:

☐ **I do not want life-sustaining treatments (including CPR) started. If life-sustaining treatments are started, I want them Stopped.**

☐ **I want life-sustaining treatments that my doctors think are best for me.**

☐ **Other wishes:** ______________________________
____
____
____
____
____
____
____
____
____

Living Will

Artificial Nutrition and Hydration

☐ **I do not want artificial nutrition started if it would be the main treatment keeping me alive. If artificial nutrition is started, I want it stopped.**

☐ **I do not want artificial hydration started if it would be the main treatment keeping me alive. If artificial hydration is started, I want it stopped.**

☐ **I want artificial nutrition even if it is the main treatment keeping me alive.**

☐ **I want artificial hydration even if it is the main treatment keeping me alive.**

☐ **Other wishes:** ______________________________

____

____

____

____

____

____

____

____

____

Living Will

Comfort Care

☐ I want to be kept as comfortable and free of pain as possible, even if it leads to reduced consciousness.

☐ Other wishes: ____________________

____

____

____

____

____

____

____

____

____

Other Directions:

You have the right to be involved in all decisions about medical care. If you have wishes not covered in other parts of this document, please indicate them here.

____

____

____

____

____

____

Living Will Required Signatures

Your Signature:

By my signature below, I show that I understand the purpose and the effect of this document.

Print Name: ______________________________
Signature: ______________________________
Date: ______________________________

Your Witnesses' Signature:

I believe the person who has signed this advance directive to be of sound mind, that he/she signed or acknowledged this advance directive in my presence, and that he/she appears not to be acting under pressure, duress, fraud, or undue influence.

Witness #1

Print Name: ______________________________
Signature: ______________________________
Date: ______________________________
Address: ______________________________

Witness #2

Print Name: ______________________________
Signature: ______________________________
Date: ______________________________
Address: ______________________________
____

Organ donation

☐ **I want to donate all my organs and tissues.**

☐ **I only want to donate these organs and tissues:__**

____

____

____

____

____

____

____

____

____

☐ **I do not wish to donate any of my organs and tissues.**

☐ **Other wishes:** ________________

____

____

____

____

____

____

____

____

____

Print Name: ______________________________

Signature: ______________________________

Date: ______________________________

Durable Power of Attorney

I appoint this person to make decisions about my medical care if there ever comes a time when I cannot make those decisions myself:

Name: ______________________________
Home Phone: _________________________
Work Phone: __________________________
Address: _______________________________
____

If the person I appointed first cannot or will not make decisions for me, I appoint this person:

Name: ______________________________
Home Phone: _________________________
Work Phone: __________________________
Address: _______________________________
____

I have not appointed anyone to make health care decisions for me in any other documents.

Signature: ____

Date: ____

Witness: ____

Date: ____

DO NOT RESUSCITATE ORDER

I request that in the event my heart and breathing should stop, no person shall attempt to resuscitate me.

This order is effective until it is revoked by me.

Being of sound mind, I voluntarily execute this order, and I understand its full import.

____

(Declarant's signature and Date)

____

(Print Declarant's full name)

____

(Signature of person who signed for declarant, if applicable and Date)

____

(Print full name)

ATTESTATION OF WITNESS

The individual who has executed this order appears to be of sound mind, and under no duress, fraud, or undue influence. Upon executing this order, the individual has (has not) received an identification bracelet.

____

(Witness signature and Date)

____

(Print witness's name)

Notary Stamp Here:

LIMITED RESUSCITATE ORDER

The physician must indicate, by checking below, those interventions to be used

_____ **Pulmonary ventilation (Resuscitation mask or ambu bag)**

_____ **Intubation**

_____ **Cardiac Massage**

_____ **Insertion of temporary pacemaker wires**

_____ **External pacemaker**

_____ **Central Lines**

_____ **Medication**

__________ ______________________________

Date **Signature of Attending Physician**

Notes: